Cobenfy

A New Hope for Schizophrenia Patients"

DR. Rebekah M. Williams

Copyright © [2024]

All rights reserved. No part of this book may be reproduced, distributed, or transmitted in any form or by any means, including photocopying, recording, or other electronic or mechanical methods, without the prior written permission of the publisher, except in the case of brief quotations embodied in critical reviews and certain other noncommercial uses permitted by copyright law.

Table of Contents

Introduction
Overview of Schizophrenia and its Treatment
CHAPTER 1
Understanding the mechanism of action of Cobenfy
FDA Approval and Regulatory Status
Comparative Effectiveness with Other Antipsychotics

CHAPTER 2
Cobenfy in Clinical Practice(Dosage and administration)
Efficacy and Safety in Different Patient Populations
Comparative Effectiveness with Other Antipsychotics

CHAPTER 3
Cobenfy: A Closer Look (Potential Benefits and Advantages)
Future Research Directions and Developments

Conclusion
Summary of key findings and insights(Future perspectives and potential impact)
Future Perspectives and Potential Impact
Recommendations for Further Research and Clinical Practice

Appendices
Detailed Information on Clinical Trials

Introduction

Overview of Schizophrenia and its Treatment

Schizophrenia is a severe and persistent mental disorder that impacts around one percent of the world's population. Cognitive deficits, disordered thought processes, hallucinations, and delusions are some of the symptoms. Social disengagement, decreased communication, and lower motivation are some of how these symptoms greatly affect a person's capacity to operate in everyday life.

Antipsychotic drugs that act on brain dopamine receptors have long been the mainstay of schizophrenia treatment. The introduction of medications like haloperidol and chlorpromazine in the middle of the twentieth century completely changed the face of mental health treatment by addressing psychotic symptoms like delusions and hallucinations. Improved symptom management with fewer side effects was achieved with the development of second-generation antipsychotics, such as risperidone and olanzapine, throughout the years.

Although there have been advancements, conventional antipsychotics still have their limits. Although they help with psychosis, they don't always help with the negative and cognitive symptoms of schizophrenia, such as being socially isolated, unmotivated, and having trouble organizing one's ideas. Moreover, the long-term use of dopamine antagonists is associated with substantial adverse effects, including weight gain, metabolic syndrome, and mobility difficulties. Consequently, there is an increasing demand for innovative treatment solutions that provide superior results for patients.

A New Era in Treatment Choices

In the hunt for more effective medicines, research has focused on uncovering alternative pathways in the brain that may be implicated in schizophrenia. One of the most encouraging advances has been the approval of Cobenfy, a first-in-class medication that targets muscarinic receptors rather than dopamine receptors. This novel method of treatment offers a significant advance, bringing hope to patients who have not reacted well to standard medicine.

Cobenfy's mode of action is radically different from prior antipsychotic medications. By regulating muscarinic receptors in the brain, notably the M1 and M4 subtypes, Cobenfy provides a unique strategy to address both the psychotic and cognitive symptoms of schizophrenia. This makes it an intriguing choice for those who struggle with the adverse effects and limitations of dopamine-based therapy.

The approval of Cobenfy signals a turning point in the treatment of schizophrenia. For the first time in decades, there is a breakthrough medicine that may give improved results for persons with this severe mental condition. This discovery not only emphasizes the significance of continuous innovation in mental treatment but also provides renewed optimism to patients and healthcare professionals alike.

The Evolution of Schizophrenia Treatments
For decades, the core of schizophrenia therapy has focused on dopamine receptor antagonists. The development of these drugs in the 1950s heralded a breakthrough in controlling psychosis since they primarily targeted dopamine D2 receptors to decrease the positive symptoms of schizophrenia, such as hallucinations and delusions. These first-generation antipsychotics, including medications like chlorpromazine and haloperidol, changed psychiatric treatment by lowering the need for long-term institutionalization of patients.

However, these medications were not without their disadvantages. Their success in treating positive sensations was countered by significant adverse effects, including extrapyramidal symptoms (EPS), which might emerge as involuntary movements or tremors. The emergence of second-generation antipsychotics (SGAs) like risperidone and clozapine is intended to alleviate these negative effects. SGAs targeted both dopamine and serotonin receptors, enabling a broader spectrum of symptom management with a lower risk of EPS.

Despite advancements, SGAs still had constraints. Many patients continued to suffer from negative and cognitive symptoms—those characteristics of schizophrenia that include social disengagement, reduced emotional expression, and difficulty with mental processing. These symptoms are very distressing, frequently leaving patients unable to lead completely productive lives, even with medication Additionally, the metabolic adverse effects associated with SGAs, such as weight gain and increased risk for diabetes, further limited their usage.

The Search for Novel Treatments

As the limits of dopamine-based therapy became increasingly evident, the focus of schizophrenia research began to shift. Scientists studied different neurotransmitter systems that may be implicated in the sickness. One interesting path of investigation was the cholinergic system, notably the muscarinic receptors in the brain, which are involved in cognition, memory, and perception. This led to the discovery of Cobenfy, a medication that targets muscarinic receptors, giving an altogether new strategy for treating schizophrenia.

Cobenfy combines xanomeline, a muscarinic receptor agonist, with trospium chloride, a peripheral muscarinic antagonist. Xanomeline preferentially activates M1 and M4 receptors in the brain, which are considered to play a role in cognitive functioning and psychosis. Trospium chloride, on the other hand, mitigates peripheral side effects by inhibiting muscarinic receptors outside the brain.

This novel approach constitutes a paradigm shift in the treatment of schizophrenia, as Cobenfy does not directly interact with dopamine receptors. Instead, it exploits a whole separate neurotransmitter system, giving a fresh alternative for patients who have not received relief with standard therapy. The findings from the EMERGENT clinical studies have demonstrated encouraging decreases in both positive and negative symptoms, making Cobenfy a milestone in the sector.

CHAPTER 1

Understanding the mechanism of action of Cobenfy

The Mechanism of Action of Cobenfy
Cobenfy (xanomeline and trospium chloride) functions through a novel method of action that distinguishes it from other antipsychotics. Unlike other schizophrenia therapies that predominantly target dopamine receptors, Cobenfy concentrates on muscarinic acetylcholine receptors (M1 and M4 subtypes) in the brain. This specific muscarinic agonism plays a vital role in regulating cognitive processes and reducing both the positive and negative symptoms of schizophrenia.

Xanomeline, the primary component of Cobenfy, operates as an agonist of the muscarinic receptors, impacting cognitive activities including attention, learning, and memory. These regions are significant, since they typically stay impaired in people with schizophrenia, even after other symptoms are controlled By activating these receptors, Cobenfy helps both the psychotic and cognitive components of schizophrenia without affecting dopamine pathways. This is a critical step forward, as it avoids many of the frequent adverse effects of standard antipsychotics, such as extrapyramidal symptoms and tardive dyskinesia.

Trospium chloride, the second component of Cobenfy, is added to minimize the peripheral adverse effects generated by xanomeline's activation of muscarinic receptors outside the brain. It suppresses muscarinic receptors in peripheral tissues, reducing undesirable effects such as gastrointestinal difficulties and cardiovascular symptoms

Chemical Structure and Pharmacological Properties

Cobenfy is composed of two active molecules: xanomeline and trospium chloride. Xanomeline is a muscarinic receptor agonist with a specific affinity for the M1 and M4 subtypes. This molecule's unique pharmacology enables it to impact brain circuits involved in cognition and psychosisl. It skips dopamine receptors, which have traditionally been the principal focus of schizophrenia therapy.

Trospium chloride, an antimuscarinic drug, does not pass the blood-brain barrier and is used to prevent the systemic adverse effects associated with xanomeline. By acting on peripheral receptors, trospium chloride lowers difficulties such as elevated heart rate, urine retention, and gastrointestinal discomfort[8†source

This combination of central muscarinic activation and peripheral muscarinic blocking leads to a medication that can target brain areas involved in schizophrenia while reducing undesired effects elsewhere in the body.

Development and Clinical Trials

The creation of Cobenfy represents decades of study into other neurotransmitter systems beyond dopamine. Early research on muscarinic receptor agonists began with xanomeline, which first showed promise in treating Alzheimer's disease. However, considerable peripheral side effects impeded its continued development for that purpose Researchers next turned to schizophrenia, an area in severe need of fresh therapeutic options, particularly for tackling cognitive deficiencies.

Cobenfy's effectiveness was proven in the EMERGENT-2 and EMERGENT-3 Phase III clinical trials. These studies comprised people with schizophrenia who were randomized to receive either Cobenfy or a placebo. The results were extremely significant, with Cobenfy demonstrating decreases in the Positive and Negative Syndrome Scale (PANSS) ratings by 9.6 and 8.4 points in the two trials, respectively. These studies indicated Cobenfy's potential to cure not just psychotic symptoms but also cognitive deficits, giving total symptom alleviation.

Additionally, Cobenfy satisfied secondary goals in these studies, such as improvements in the Clinical Global Impression-Severity (CGI-S) ratings, further solidifying its efficacy in schizophrenia treatment The drug's safety profile was also investigated in long-term open-label studies, which indicated that patients tolerated Cobenfy well over longer durations, with controllable side effects such as dry mouth, constipation, and moderate cardiovascular symptoms.

FDA Approval and Regulatory Status

On September 27, 2024, the FDA awarded clearance to Cobenfy, making it the first new class of schizophrenia medication in several decades【9†source】. This approval was based on the compelling findings from the EMERGENT studies, which confirmed Cobenfy's effectiveness and safety profile. With its unique method targeting muscarinic receptors, the medication marks a substantial advance in neuropsychiatry.

The approval of Cobenfy signified a dramatic change in the regulatory environment for schizophrenia medicines. After decades of depending on dopamine-modulating medicines, the discovery of a therapy that exploits an entirely other neurotransmitter system marks a new era of therapeutic options. The FDA's decision was viewed as a milestone for both the scientific community and patients since it widened the choices for people who had previously been confined to dopamine-based treatments

Beyond the United States, Cobenfy is scheduled to face regulatory evaluations in Europe, Asia, and other areas, thereby widening its effect on global mental health treatment. Its approval has prompted expectations that other innovative, receptor-specific medications may follow, allowing patients a greater choice of therapeutic options in the future.

This chapter gives a detailed look at Cobenfy's pharmacology, its development via clinical trials, and its relevance as a revolutionary therapy for schizophrenia.

CHAPTER 2

Cobenfy in Clinical Practice(Dosage and administration)

Dosage and Administration

Cobenfy is delivered as an oral tablet and is commonly prescribed in a fixed combination of xanomeline and trospium chloride. The normal suggested dose is 50 mg of xanomeline and 20 mg of trospium chloride, given twice a day. However, the dose may be changed based on individual patient requirements, tolerability, and response to treatment. It's vital to remember that Cobenfy should be taken with meals to optimize absorption and decrease gastrointestinal adverse effects.

In clinical practice, titration to the maximum therapeutic dose is typically suggested throughout the first week of treatment to allow the body to adjust to the medicine. Patients starting Cobenfy may encounter modest side effects during this period, which normally decrease as the body adjusts.

Monitoring and Management of Side Effects
While Cobenfy has been demonstrated to be generally well tolerated, physicians must monitor patients for any adverse effects. The most prevalent side effects observed throughout clinical trials were gastrointestinal, such as nausea, constipation, and dry mouth These effects are generally mild to moderate and may frequently be controlled with supportive care or dosage modifications.

Other adverse effects may include urinary retention and tachycardia, due to the muscarinic action of xanomeline. Trospium chloride, added in the formulation, helps decrease the impact of these peripheral adverse effects. In patients with a history of cardiovascular difficulties, it is crucial to constantly monitor heart rate and rhythm, particularly in the early phases of treatment

Regular follow-up visits should be made to monitor tolerance, effectiveness, and the occurrence of any side effects. Since Cobenfy is metabolized via the liver and kidneys, hepatic and renal function should be frequently monitored, especially in individuals with preexisting disorders that might impair drug clearance].

Efficacy and Safety in Different Patient Populations

Cobenfy has shown promising effectiveness across a broad spectrum of individuals with schizophrenia, including those with treatment-resistant symptoms. Clinical studies revealed statistically substantial decreases in both positive and negative symptoms of schizophrenia, notably in individuals who had not reacted well to standard dopamine-receptor antagonists

Patients with comorbid conditions such as diabetes, metabolic syndrome, or cardiovascular disease may find Cobenfy to be a preferred alternative since it does not carry the same risk of metabolic side effects seen with second-generation antipsychotics (SGAs) However, patients with significant hepatic or renal impairment may not be acceptable candidates for the

drug owing to its dependency on these organs for metabolism and disposal. Special care should be given in dosing and monitoring for these groups.

Cobenfy's unique mechanism also shows promise in younger patients with early-onset schizophrenia, giving potential advantages in cognitive and functional outcomes. However, further study is needed to completely prove its safety in pediatric groups.

Comparative Effectiveness with Other Antipsychotics

When compared to typical antipsychotics, notably first- and second-generation dopamine antagonists, Cobenfy stands apart due to its unique mode of action. Unlike standard antipsychotics, which largely operate by inhibiting dopamine D2 receptors, Cobenfy exclusively targets muscarinic receptors, giving a unique strategy to address symptoms without generating dopamine-related side effects including tardive dyskinesia or extrapyramidal symptoms (EPS)

Cobenfy also appears to have a lower risk of metabolic side effects, such as weight gain and insulin resistance, which are frequent with SGAs like olanzapine or clozapine. This makes Cobenfy a potentially safer long-term alternative, especially for those at risk of developing metabolic disorders.

In terms of effectiveness, Cobenfy has been proven to cause considerable improvements in symptomatology compared to placebo, notably in lowering negative and cognitive symptoms that are generally resistant to treatment with standard antipsychotics. Its comparative efficacy versus alternative muscarinic or glutamatergic-based medicines remains a topic of current research, but early data show that Cobenfy is a strong competitor in rethinking schizophrenia therapy.

This chapter covers Cobenfy's real-world applications, concentrating on how it integrates into clinical practice, and patient care, and its comparative benefits over conventional therapies.

CHAPTER 3

Cobenfy: A Closer Look (Potential Benefits and Advantages)

Cobenfy has numerous substantial advantages over standard antipsychotics, making it a breakthrough in schizophrenia therapy. One of its key advantages rests in its novel method of action—targeting muscarinic receptors (M1 and M4) instead of dopamine receptors. This technique allows it to treat schizophrenia without producing typical dopamine-related side effects, such as **tardive dyskinesia** or extrapyramidal symptoms (EPS), which have long been a difficulty for patients on standard antipsychotic medications. This is a crucial development for those individuals who endure terrible mobility abnormalities owing to long-term antipsychotic usage.

In addition to treating positive symptoms like hallucinations and delusions, Cobenfy has also proven efficacy in reducing negative symptoms and cognitive deficits, which are typically inadequately addressed by conventional treatments Negative symptoms, such as social disengagement and dampened effect, are key contributors to the poor quality of life in schizophrenia patients, and current treatments give minimal help for these components of the condition. Cobenfy's capacity to target muscarinic receptors, which are important in cognition, may lead to improved outcomes in areas like memory, attention, and executive function, enabling a more holistic approach to symptom management

Furthermore, Cobenfy has been proven to have fewer metabolic adverse effects compared to second-generation antipsychotics (SGAs), which are commonly linked with weight gain, insulin resistance, and an increased risk of diabetes. This makes Cobenfy a safer long-term choice, especially for individuals who are at higher risk of metabolic complications

Limitations and Challenges

Despite its advantages, Cobenfy is not without restrictions and obstacles. While the medicine is well tolerated in many situations, it is nevertheless linked with gastrointestinal side effects, such as nausea and constipation, as well as cardiovascular concerns, including tachycardia and urine retention. These adverse effects, although lessened by the addition of trospium chloride, nonetheless require cautious treatment and patient monitoring, particularly in those with prior cardiovascular issues.

Another restriction is that Cobenfy has not yet been evaluated extensively in special populations, such as pregnant or nursing women, the elderly, or persons with severe hepatic or renal impairments. These categories may require different doses or have specific dangers that have not been adequately studied in clinical trials. Furthermore, while Cobenfy has shown promise in early studies, it is a relatively new medicine, and long-term data on its efficacy and safety are still being obtained. This raises doubts regarding its longevity as a therapy option and its potential for deleterious consequences with continued usage.

Lastly, cost and accessibility may cause issues. As a novel drug, Cobenfy might be pricey and may not yet be readily accessible in all regions or covered by all insurance companies. Patients without proper health insurance may find it challenging to receive this innovative therapy, particularly in lower-income settings

Future Research Directions and Developments

The approval of Cobenfy opens the door for further research into the function of muscarinic receptors in schizophrenia and other mental diseases. Future studies will likely study its long-term effectiveness, safety, and the possibility of its usage in conjunction with other therapies. Researchers are also researching whether Cobenfy may be beneficial in treating illnesses outside schizophrenia, such as bipolar disorder or Alzheimer's disease, given its cognitive-enhancing properties

Additionally, there is considerable interest in developing **biomarkers** that might predict which patients will respond best to Cobenfy. This would allow for a more tailored approach to schizophrenia therapy, eliminating the trial-and-error process often required in identifying the proper medicine for each patient.

Ongoing research into the next generation of muscarinic receptor modulators may also deliver medications with even fewer adverse effects or higher selectivity for certain receptor subtypes, significantly enhancing the treatment landscape for mental health problems. The future of Cobenfy and comparable medicines will depend greatly on continuing clinical studies and real-world data on patient results.

Ethical Considerations and Social Implications

The introduction of Cobenfy poses various ethical considerations, notably surrounding its availability and distribution. As with every new medicine, there is a danger that its high cost may limit distribution to particular socioeconomic groups, expanding the imbalance in mental health treatment. Ensuring that Cobenfy is available to all patients, regardless of financial situation, is a crucial ethical problem that has to be addressed by both healthcare practitioners and policymakers.

There are also worries concerning the over-medicalization of psychiatric illnesses. With the debut of a new class of pharmaceuticals, there is always a fear that therapies may be overprescribed, perhaps leading to unwarranted medicalization of particular behaviors or diseases. Careful guidelines and monitoring are essential to ensure that Cobenfy is used effectively and that patients receive the most effective, evidence-based therapy.

Finally, the social implications of a novel medicine like Cobenfy are crucial. Schizophrenia bears a severe stigma, and breakthroughs in its treatment can help alleviate this stigma by portraying the condition as one with appropriate medical management choices. Improved therapies can boost patients' quality of life, increase their capacity to engage in society, and eventually contribute to lessening the marginalization commonly faced by those with severe mental illness

This chapter discusses the larger implications of Cobenfy, touching on its advantages, limits, and future paths of study, while also addressing the ethical and social problems that come with its implementation into therapeutic practice.

Conclusion

Summary of key findings and insights(Future perspectives and potential impact)

Cobenfy offers a substantial improvement in the treatment of schizophrenia, proposing a novel mechanism of action by targeting muscarinic receptors instead of the usual dopamine routes. This medicine has shown efficacy in lowering both positive and negative symptoms, coupled with cognitive deficiencies, giving comprehensive treatment for patients who have battled with traditional antipsychotics. Its ability to avoid common dopamine-related side effects, such as tardive dyskinesia and extrapyramidal symptoms, further strengthens its relevance in clinical practice. Additionally, Cobenfy appears to have a better safety profile in terms of metabolic side effects, which is critical for long-term patient results.

However, despite these benefits, there are still limitations and challenges to consider, such as the treatment of gastrointestinal and cardiovascular adverse effects, and the need for greater evidence on its long-term effectiveness and safety in varied patient populations. While Cobenfy provides a significant option for people resistant to standard therapies, additional study is necessary to address its limitations and maximize its usage in clinical practice.

Future Perspectives and Potential Impact

The launch of Cobenfy is anticipated to have a dramatic influence on the **future of schizophrenia treatment. It is the first step in a new class of medications that might change the focus away from dopamine antagonism and toward more targeted therapies based on individual neurobiological profiles. This technique offers the potential to personalize schizophrenia treatment, giving a targeted strategy that improves patient results and quality of life.

Moreover, Cobenfy's success might stimulate future research into muscarinic receptors and their function in other neuropsychiatric illnesses, such as Alzheimer's disease and bipolar disorder. approval establishes a precedent for the development of new medications that might better address the **cognitive and functional deficits** that many individuals with schizophrenia face.

Recommendations for Further Research and Clinical Practice

While Cobenfy has shown significant potential, there are some areas where additional research is essential. Long-term studies are needed to properly establish its safety profile, particularly concerning its cardiovascular effects and its usage in special populations, such as the elderly and those with comorbidities. Furthermore, research exploring the combination of Cobenfy with other therapies might give insights into how best to integrate this medicine into established treatment regimens for schizophrenia.

From a clinical standpoint, healthcare practitioners should employ comprehensive monitoring techniques to control side effects effectively and alter doses as necessary. As availability to Cobenfy develops, practitioners should also work on ensuring equitable distribution of this breakthrough medicine, ensuring that all patients, regardless of socioeconomic situation, have access to this potentially life-changing medication.

This conclusion weaves together the important results of Cobenfy's influence on schizophrenia therapy while identifying critical prospects and proposing recommendations for additional study and clinical integration.

Appendices

Detailed Information on Clinical Trials

Cobenfy has undergone extensive clinical studies, most notably the **EMERGENT-2** and **EMERGENT-3** trials, which were essential in showing its effectiveness and safety for treating schizophrenia. These trials were Phase III investigations that included double-blind, placebo-controlled procedures to assure thorough testing. Participants were randomized into two groups: those getting Cobenfy and those receiving a placebo.

Key findings from these trials include:
- decrease in PANSS Scores: Cobenfy resulted in a substantial decrease in Positive and Negative

Syndrome Scale (PANSS) scores, with reductions of 9.6 and 8.4 points, respectively, in the two trials- Secondary Endpoints: Improvements were also seen in Clinical Global Impression-Severity (CGI-S) ratings, confirming Cobenfy's comprehensive influence on symptom severity.
- Safety Profile: The studies showed tolerable side effects, including gastrointestinal difficulties (nausea, constipation) and cardiovascular symptoms including tachycardia, which were handled with trospium chloride.

For more extensive information, clinical trial data may be accessible through sites like **ClinicalTrials.gov** under the identifiers **NCT03952486** and **NCT04224413**, or through the FDA drug approval documentation.

Patient Resources and Support Organizations
Living with schizophrenia can be tough, but several organizations give vital services and support:

- National Alliance on Mental Illness (NAMI): NAMI offers support groups, educational resources, and advocacy activities for persons living with schizophrenia and their families. Their hotline is accessible for rapid support and consultation. [Website: nami.org](https://www.nami.org)

- **Schizophrenia & Psychosis Action Alliance (S&PAA)**: This organization focuses on increasing the research, treatment, and care for persons with schizophrenia. They also offer peer-led support groups and lobbying for improved mental health treatment. [Website: section.org](https://www.sczaction.org)

-**Mental Health America (MHA):** MHA provides materials relating to mental health education, early intervention, and advocacy. They provide online screening tools for mental health conditions and connections to local support resources. [Website: mhanational.org](https://www.mhanational.org)

Glossary of Terms

- **Muscarinic Receptors:** A kind of acetylcholine receptor implicated in several brain functions, including cognition, memory, and psychosis. Cobenfy particularly targets **M1 and M4** receptors to relieve schizophrenia symptoms.
- **Positive Symptoms:** Schizophrenia symptoms include hallucinations, delusions, and disordered thinking. These are generally the most noticeable and disruptive symptoms.
- **Negative Symptoms:** These pertain to emotional and social retreat, lack of drive, and a flattened affect. Negative symptoms are less responsive to typical antipsychotic therapies but are addressed by Cobenfy.
- **PANSS (Positive and Negative Syndrome Scale):** A medical scale used to quantify the severity of schizophrenia symptoms. It analyzes positive, negative, and general psychopathological symptoms.
- **CGI-S (Clinical Global Impression-Severity):** A clinician-rated scale that evaluates the overall severity of mental illness based on observed behavior and patient self-reports.

- **Extrapyramidal Symptoms (EPS)**: Movement abnormalities produced by dopamine-blocking medications, include tremors, rigidity, and tardive dyskinesia. These side effects are not prevalent with Cobenfy due to its non-dopaminergic action.

The End

www.ingramcontent.com/pod-product-compliance
Lightning Source LLC
LaVergne TN
LVHW021450231224
799792LV00005B/492